This Journal Belongs To

Medical Disclaimer:

The information included in this book is for educational purposes only. It is not intended or implied to be a substitute for professional medical advice, diagnosis, or treatment. The reader should always consult with her or his health care provider before beginning a new health care regimen or weight loss program.

My Journey

Start Day

_____

Personal Goals

_____

_____

_____

_____

_____

_____

_____

Why is this goal important for me to accomplish?
How will it change my health and my life?

_____

_____

_____

_____

_____

_____

_____

_____

_____

_____

_____

_____

_____

_____

_____

_____

Progress Tracker

Date [   ]

	Measurement	Loss / Gain
Weight		
Left Arm		
Right Arm		
Chest		
Waist		
Hips		
Left Thigh		
Right Thigh		

Weekly Goals

[   ]

How are you feeling at the beginning of your first week?

_____

_____

_____

_____

_____

_____

_____

_____

_____

_____

_____

_____

_____

_____

_____

_____

Date	Day of Week	Weight

Breakfast

Time _____   Rate your Hunger 1-10 _____

_____

_____

Lunch

Time _____   Rate your Hunger 1-10 _____

_____

_____

Dinner

Time _____   Rate your Hunger 1-10 _____

_____

_____

Snacks

Time _____

Why am I eating this snack?

_____

Time _____

Why am I eating this snack?

_____

Water ⬤ 8oz ◯ ◯ ◯ ◯ ◯ ◯ ◯

Beverages

_____

_____

Cravings / Responses

_____

_____

Activity / Exercise

_____

_____

How to make tomorrow better

_____

_____

_____

_____

I am so proud of myself today because I...

_____

_____

_____

_____

Date	Day of Week	Weight

Breakfast

Time _____   Rate your Hunger 1-10 _____

_____

_____

Lunch

Time _____   Rate your Hunger 1-10 _____

_____

_____

Dinner

Time _____   Rate your Hunger 1-10 _____

_____

_____

Snacks

Time _____

Why am I eating this snack?

_____

Time _____

Why am I eating this snack?

_____

Water ⬤ 8oz ◯ ◯ ◯ ◯ ◯ ◯ ◯ ◯

Beverages

_____

_____

Cravings / Responses

_____

_____

Activity / Exercise

_____

_____

How to make tomorrow better

_____

_____

_____

_____

I am so proud of myself today because I...

_____

_____

_____

_____

Date	Day of Week	Weight

Breakfast

Time _____   Rate your Hunger 1-10 _____

_____

_____

Lunch

Time _____   Rate your Hunger 1-10 _____

_____

_____

Dinner

Time _____   Rate your Hunger 1-10 _____

_____

_____

Snacks

Time _____

Why am I eating this snack?

_____

Time _____

Why am I eating this snack?

_____

Water ⬡ 8oz ◯ ◯ ◯ ◯ ◯ ◯ ◯

Beverages

_____

_____

Cravings / Responses

_____

_____

Activity / Exercise

_____

_____

How to make tomorrow better

_____

_____

_____

_____

I am so proud of myself today because I...

_____

_____

_____

_____

Date	Day of Week	Weight

Breakfast

Time _____   Rate your Hunger 1-10 _____

_____

_____

Lunch

Time _____   Rate your Hunger 1-10 _____

_____

_____

Dinner

Time _____   Rate your Hunger 1-10 _____

_____

_____

Snacks

Time _____

Why am I eating this snack?

_____

Time _____

Why am I eating this snack?

_____

Water 🜄 8oz ○ ○ ○ ○ ○ ○ ○

Beverages

_____

_____

Cravings / Responses

_____

_____

Activity / Exercise

_____

_____

How to make tomorrow better

_____

_____

_____

_____

I am so proud of myself today because I...

_____

_____

_____

_____

Date	Day of Week	Weight

Breakfast

Time _____   Rate your Hunger 1-10 _____

_____

_____

Lunch

Time _____   Rate your Hunger 1-10 _____

_____

_____

Dinner

Time _____   Rate your Hunger 1-10 _____

_____

_____

Snacks

Time _____

Why am I eating this snack?

_____

Time _____

Why am I eating this snack?

_____

Water ⬦ 8oz ◯ ◯ ◯ ◯ ◯ ◯ ◯

Beverages

_____

_____

Cravings / Responses

_____

_____

Activity / Exercise

_____

_____

How to make tomorrow better

_____

_____

_____

_____

I am so proud of myself today because I...

_____

_____

_____

_____

Date

Day of Week

Weight

Breakfast

Time _____

Rate your Hunger 1-10 _____

_____

_____

Lunch

Time _____

Rate your Hunger 1-10 _____

_____

_____

Dinner

Time _____

Rate your Hunger 1-10 _____

_____

_____

Snacks

Time _____

Why am I eating this snack?

_____

Time _____

Why am I eating this snack?

_____

Water ⬤ 8oz ◯ ◯ ◯ ◯ ◯ ◯ ◯

Beverages

_____

_____

Cravings / Responses

_____

_____

Activity / Exercise

_____

_____

How to make tomorrow better

_____

_____

_____

_____

I am so proud of myself today because I...

_____

_____

_____

_____

Date	Day of Week	Weight

Breakfast

Time _____   Rate your Hunger 1-10 _____

_____

_____

Lunch

Time _____   Rate your Hunger 1-10 _____

_____

_____

Dinner

Time _____   Rate your Hunger 1-10 _____

_____

_____

Snacks

Time _____

Why am I eating this snack?

_____

Time _____

Why am I eating this snack?

_____

Water 🌢 8oz ◯ ◯ ◯ ◯ ◯ ◯ ◯

Beverages

_____

_____

Cravings / Responses

_____

_____

Activity / Exercise

_____

_____

How to make tomorrow better

_____

_____

_____

_____

I am so proud of myself today because I...

_____

_____

_____

_____

Weekly Progress Tracker

Date [   ]

	Measurement	Loss / Gain
Weight		
Left Arm		
Right Arm		
Chest		
Waist		
Hips		
Left Thigh		
Right Thigh		

Weekly Goals

What was my biggest accomplishment for the week?

_____

_____

What new healthy eating choices did I make this week?

_____

_____

What new healthy lifestyle choices did I make this week?

_____

_____

On a scale of 1 - 10 how do I feel about my health and happiness this week? Why do I feel that way?

_____

_____

_____

Rewards for pounds lost

_____

Reasons why being healthy and losing weight matters to me

_____

_____

Date	Day of Week	Weight

Breakfast

Time _____   Rate your Hunger 1-10 _____

_____

_____

Lunch

Time _____   Rate your Hunger 1-10 _____

_____

_____

Dinner

Time _____   Rate your Hunger 1-10 _____

_____

_____

Snacks

Time _____

Why am I eating this snack?

_____

Time _____

Why am I eating this snack?

_____

Water ⬡ 8oz ◯ ◯ ◯ ◯ ◯ ◯ ◯

Beverages

_____

_____

Cravings / Responses

_____

_____

Activity / Exercise

_____

_____

How to make tomorrow better

_____

_____

_____

_____

I am so proud of myself today because I...

_____

_____

_____

_____

Date	Day of Week	Weight

Breakfast

Time _____   Rate your Hunger 1-10 _____

_____

_____

Lunch

Time _____   Rate your Hunger 1-10 _____

_____

_____

Dinner

Time _____   Rate your Hunger 1-10 _____

_____

_____

Snacks

Time _____

Why am I eating this snack?

_____

Time _____

Why am I eating this snack?

_____

Water ⬦ 8oz ◯ ◯ ◯ ◯ ◯ ◯ ◯

Beverages

_____

_____

Cravings / Responses

_____

_____

Activity / Exercise

_____

_____

How to make tomorrow better

_____

_____

_____

_____

I am so proud of myself today because I...

_____

_____

_____

_____

Date _____ Day of Week _____ Weight _____

Breakfast

Time _____   Rate your Hunger 1-10 _____

_____

_____

Lunch

Time _____   Rate your Hunger 1-10 _____

_____

_____

Dinner

Time _____   Rate your Hunger 1-10 _____

_____

_____

Snacks

Time _____

Why am I eating this snack?

_____

Time _____

Why am I eating this snack?

_____

Water ○ 8oz ◯ ◯ ◯ ◯ ◯ ◯ ◯

Beverages

_____

_____

Cravings / Responses

_____

_____

Activity / Exercise

_____

_____

How to make tomorrow better

_____

_____

_____

_____

I am so proud of myself today because I...

_____

_____

_____

_____

Date	Day of Week	Weight

Breakfast

Time _____   Rate your Hunger 1-10 _____

_____

_____

Lunch

Time _____   Rate your Hunger 1-10 _____

_____

_____

Dinner

Time _____   Rate your Hunger 1-10 _____

_____

_____

Snacks

Time _____

Why am I eating this snack?

_____

Time _____

Why am I eating this snack?

_____

Water ⬭ 8oz ○ ○ ○ ○ ○ ○ ○ ○

Beverages

_____

_____

Cravings / Responses

_____

_____

Activity / Exercise

_____

_____

How to make tomorrow better

_____

_____

_____

_____

I am so proud of myself today because I...

_____

_____

_____

_____

Date	Day of Week	Weight

Breakfast

Time _____   Rate your Hunger 1-10 _____

_____

_____

Lunch

Time _____   Rate your Hunger 1-10 _____

_____

_____

Dinner

Time _____   Rate your Hunger 1-10 _____

_____

_____

Snacks

Time _____

Why am I eating this snack?

_____

Time _____

Why am I eating this snack?

_____

Water ⬦ 8oz ◯ ◯ ◯ ◯ ◯ ◯ ◯

Beverages

_____

_____

Cravings / Responses

_____

_____

Activity / Exercise

_____

_____

How to make tomorrow better

_____

_____

_____

_____

I am so proud of myself today because I...

_____

_____

_____

_____

Date	Day of Week	Weight

Breakfast

Time _____   Rate your Hunger 1-10 _____

_____

_____

Lunch

Time _____   Rate your Hunger 1-10 _____

_____

_____

Dinner

Time _____   Rate your Hunger 1-10 _____

_____

_____

Snacks

Time _____

Why am I eating this snack?

_____

Time _____

Why am I eating this snack?

_____

Water ⬭ 8oz ○ ○ ○ ○ ○ ○ ○

Beverages

_____

_____

Cravings / Responses

_____

_____

Activity / Exercise

_____

_____

How to make tomorrow better

_____

_____

_____

_____

I am so proud of myself today because I...

_____

_____

_____

_____

Date	Day of Week	Weight

Breakfast

Time _____   Rate your Hunger 1-10 _____

_____

_____

Lunch

Time _____   Rate your Hunger 1-10 _____

_____

_____

Dinner

Time _____   Rate your Hunger 1-10 _____

_____

_____

Snacks

Time _____

Why am I eating this snack?

_____

Time _____

Why am I eating this snack?

_____

Water ⬡ 8oz ◯ ◯ ◯ ◯ ◯ ◯ ◯

Beverages

_____

_____

Cravings / Responses

_____

_____

Activity / Exercise

_____

_____

How to make tomorrow better

_____

_____

_____

_____

I am so proud of myself today because I...

_____

_____

_____

_____

Weekly Progress Tracker

Date [_____]

	Measurement	Loss / Gain
Weight		
Left Arm		
Right Arm		
Chest		
Waist		
Hips		
Left Thigh		
Right Thigh		

Weekly Goals

What was my biggest accomplishment for the week?

_____

_____

What new healthy eating choices did I make this week?

_____

_____

What new healthy lifestyle choices did I make this week?

_____

_____

On a scale of 1 - 10 how do I feel about my health and happiness this week? Why do I feel that way?

_____

_____

_____

Rewards for pounds lost

_____

Reasons why being healthy and losing weight matters to me

_____

_____

Date	Day of Week	Weight

Breakfast

Time _____   Rate your Hunger 1-10 _____

_____

_____

Lunch

Time _____   Rate your Hunger 1-10 _____

_____

_____

Dinner

Time _____   Rate your Hunger 1-10 _____

_____

_____

Snacks

Time _____

Why am I eating this snack?

_____

Time _____

Why am I eating this snack?

_____

Water ◯ 8oz ◯ ◯ ◯ ◯ ◯ ◯ ◯

Beverages

_____

_____

Cravings / Responses

_____

_____

Activity / Exercise

_____

_____

How to make tomorrow better

_____

_____

_____

_____

I am so proud of myself today because I...

_____

_____

_____

_____

Date	Day of Week	Weight

Breakfast

Time _____   Rate your Hunger 1-10 _____

_____

_____

Lunch

Time _____   Rate your Hunger 1-10 _____

_____

_____

Dinner

Time _____   Rate your Hunger 1-10 _____

_____

_____

Snacks

Time _____

Why am I eating this snack?

_____

Time _____

Why am I eating this snack?

_____

Water ⬭ 8oz ◯ ◯ ◯ ◯ ◯ ◯ ◯ ◯

Beverages

_____

_____

Cravings / Responses

_____

_____

Activity / Exercise

_____

_____

How to make tomorrow better

_____

_____

_____

_____

I am so proud of myself today because I...

_____

_____

_____

_____

Date	Day of Week	Weight

Breakfast

Time _____   Rate your Hunger 1-10 _____

_____

_____

Lunch

Time _____   Rate your Hunger 1-10 _____

_____

_____

Dinner

Time _____   Rate your Hunger 1-10 _____

_____

_____

Snacks

Time _____

Why am I eating this snack?

_____

Time _____

Why am I eating this snack?

_____

Water ⬠ 8oz   ○ ○ ○ ○ ○ ○ ○ ○

Beverages

_____

_____

Cravings / Responses

_____

_____

Activity / Exercise

_____

_____

How to make tomorrow better

_____

_____

_____

_____

I am so proud of myself today because I...

_____

_____

_____

_____

Date	Day of Week	Weight

Breakfast

Time _____   Rate your Hunger 1-10 _____

_____

_____

Lunch

Time _____   Rate your Hunger 1-10 _____

_____

_____

Dinner

Time _____   Rate your Hunger 1-10 _____

_____

_____

Snacks

Time _____

Why am I eating this snack?

_____

Time _____

Why am I eating this snack?

_____

Water 💧 8oz   ⃝ ⃝ ⃝ ⃝ ⃝ ⃝ ⃝

Beverages

_____

_____

Cravings / Responses

_____

_____

Activity / Exercise

_____

_____

How to make tomorrow better

_____

_____

_____

_____

I am so proud of myself today because I...

_____

_____

_____

_____

Date	Day of Week	Weight

Breakfast

Time _____   Rate your Hunger 1-10 _____

_____

_____

Lunch

Time _____   Rate your Hunger 1-10 _____

_____

_____

Dinner

Time _____   Rate your Hunger 1-10 _____

_____

_____

Snacks

Time _____

Why am I eating this snack?

_____

Time _____

Why am I eating this snack?

_____

Water ⬤ 8oz ◯ ◯ ◯ ◯ ◯ ◯ ◯

Beverages

_____

_____

Cravings / Responses

_____

_____

Activity / Exercise

_____

_____

How to make tomorrow better

_____

_____

_____

_____

I am so proud of myself today because I...

_____

_____

_____

_____

Date	Day of Week	Weight

Breakfast

Time _____   Rate your Hunger 1-10 _____

_____

_____

Lunch

Time _____   Rate your Hunger 1-10 _____

_____

_____

Dinner

Time _____   Rate your Hunger 1-10 _____

_____

_____

Snacks

Time _____

Why am I eating this snack?

_____

Time _____

Why am I eating this snack?

_____

Water ⬤ 8oz ◯ ◯ ◯ ◯ ◯ ◯ ◯

Beverages

_____

_____

Cravings / Responses

_____

_____

Activity / Exercise

_____

_____

How to make tomorrow better

_____

_____

_____

_____

I am so proud of myself today because I...

_____

_____

_____

_____

Date	Day of Week	Weight

Breakfast

Time _____   Rate your Hunger 1-10 _____

_____

_____

Lunch

Time _____   Rate your Hunger 1-10 _____

_____

_____

Dinner

Time _____   Rate your Hunger 1-10 _____

_____

_____

Snacks

Time _____

Why am I eating this snack?

_____

Time _____

Why am I eating this snack?

_____

Water ⬡ 8oz ◯ ◯ ◯ ◯ ◯ ◯ ◯

Beverages

_____

_____

Cravings / Responses

_____

_____

Activity / Exercise

_____

_____

How to make tomorrow better

_____

_____

_____

_____

I am so proud of myself today because I...

_____

_____

_____

_____

Weekly Progress Tracker

Date [   ]

	Measurement	Loss / Gain
Weight		
Left Arm		
Right Arm		
Chest		
Waist		
Hips		
Left Thigh		
Right Thigh		

Weekly Goals

What was my biggest accomplishment for the week?

_____

_____

What new healthy eating choices did I make this week?

_____

_____

What new healthy lifestyle choices did I make this week?

_____

_____

On a scale of 1 - 10 how do I feel about my health and happiness this week? Why do I feel that way?

_____

_____

_____

Rewards for pounds lost

_____

Reasons why being healthy and losing weight matters to me

_____

_____

Date	Day of Week	Weight

Breakfast

Time _____   Rate your Hunger 1-10 _____

_____

_____

Lunch

Time _____   Rate your Hunger 1-10 _____

_____

_____

Dinner

Time _____   Rate your Hunger 1-10 _____

_____

_____

Snacks

Time _____

Why am I eating this snack?

_____

Time _____

Why am I eating this snack?

_____

Water ⬦ 8oz ◯ ◯ ◯ ◯ ◯ ◯ ◯ ◯

Beverages

_____

_____

Cravings / Responses

_____

_____

Activity / Exercise

_____

_____

How to make tomorrow better

_____

_____

_____

_____

I am so proud of myself today because I...

_____

_____

_____

_____

Date	Day of Week	Weight

Breakfast

Time _____   Rate your Hunger 1-10 _____

_____

_____

Lunch

Time _____   Rate your Hunger 1-10 _____

_____

_____

Dinner

Time _____   Rate your Hunger 1-10 _____

_____

_____

Snacks

Time _____

Why am I eating this snack?

_____

Time _____

Why am I eating this snack?

_____

Water 💧 8oz ◯ ◯ ◯ ◯ ◯ ◯ ◯

Beverages

_____

_____

Cravings / Responses

_____

_____

Activity / Exercise

_____

_____

How to make tomorrow better

_____

_____

_____

_____

I am so proud of myself today because I...

_____

_____

_____

_____

Date

[   ]

Day of Week

[   ]

Weight

[   ]

Breakfast

Time _____   Rate your Hunger 1-10 _____

_____

_____

Lunch

Time _____   Rate your Hunger 1-10 _____

_____

_____

Dinner

Time _____   Rate your Hunger 1-10 _____

_____

_____

Snacks

Time _____

Why am I eating this snack?

_____

Time _____

Why am I eating this snack?

_____

Water ⬭ 8oz ◯ ◯ ◯ ◯ ◯ ◯ ◯ ◯

Beverages

_____

_____

Cravings / Responses

_____

_____

Activity / Exercise

_____

_____

How to make tomorrow better

_____

_____

_____

_____

I am so proud of myself today because I...

_____

_____

_____

_____

Date	Day of Week	Weight

Breakfast

Time _____   Rate your Hunger 1-10 _____

_____

_____

Lunch

Time _____   Rate your Hunger 1-10 _____

_____

_____

Dinner

Time _____   Rate your Hunger 1-10 _____

_____

_____

Snacks

Time _____

Why am I eating this snack?

_____

Time _____

Why am I eating this snack?

_____

Water ⬡ 8oz ◯ ◯ ◯ ◯ ◯ ◯ ◯ ◯

Beverages

_____

_____

Cravings / Responses

_____

_____

Activity / Exercise

_____

_____

How to make tomorrow better

_____

_____

_____

_____

I am so proud of myself today because I...

_____

_____

_____

_____

Date

Day of Week

Weight

Breakfast

Time _____   Rate your Hunger 1-10 _____

_____

_____

Lunch

Time _____   Rate your Hunger 1-10 _____

_____

_____

Dinner

Time _____   Rate your Hunger 1-10 _____

_____

_____

Snacks

Time _____

Why am I eating this snack?

_____

Time _____

Why am I eating this snack?

_____

Water ○ 8oz   ○ ○ ○ ○ ○ ○ ○

Beverages

_____

_____

Cravings / Responses

_____

_____

Activity / Exercise

_____

_____

How to make tomorrow better

_____

_____

_____

_____

I am so proud of myself today because I...

_____

_____

_____

_____

Date	Day of Week	Weight

Breakfast

Time _____   Rate your Hunger 1-10 _____

_____

_____

Lunch

Time _____   Rate your Hunger 1-10 _____

_____

_____

Dinner

Time _____   Rate your Hunger 1-10 _____

_____

_____

Snacks

Time _____

Why am I eating this snack?

_____

Time _____

Why am I eating this snack?

_____

Water ⬭ 8oz ○ ○ ○ ○ ○ ○ ○

Beverages

_____

_____

Cravings / Responses

_____

_____

Activity / Exercise

_____

_____

How to make tomorrow better

_____

_____

_____

_____

I am so proud of myself today because I...

_____

_____

_____

_____

Date	Day of Week	Weight

Breakfast

Time _____   Rate your Hunger 1-10 _____

_____

_____

Lunch

Time _____   Rate your Hunger 1-10 _____

_____

_____

Dinner

Time _____   Rate your Hunger 1-10 _____

_____

_____

Snacks

Time _____

Why am I eating this snack?

_____

Time _____

Why am I eating this snack?

_____

Water ⬡ 8oz ◯ ◯ ◯ ◯ ◯ ◯ ◯ ◯

Beverages

_____

_____

Cravings / Responses

_____

_____

Activity / Exercise

_____

_____

How to make tomorrow better

_____

_____

_____

_____

I am so proud of myself today because I...

_____

_____

_____

_____

Weekly Progress Tracker

Date

	Measurement	Loss / Gain
Weight		
Left Arm		
Right Arm		
Chest		
Waist		
Hips		
Left Thigh		
Right Thigh		

Weekly Goals

What was my biggest accomplishment for the week?

_____

_____

What new healthy eating choices did I make this week?

_____

_____

What new healthy lifestyle choices did I make this week?

_____

_____

On a scale of 1 - 10 how do I feel about my health and happiness this week? Why do I feel that way?

_____

_____

_____

Rewards for pounds lost

_____

Reasons why being healthy and losing weight matters to me

_____

_____

Date

Day of Week

Weight

Breakfast

Time _____   Rate your Hunger 1-10 _____

_____

_____

Lunch

Time _____   Rate your Hunger 1-10 _____

_____

_____

Dinner

Time _____   Rate your Hunger 1-10 _____

_____

_____

Snacks

Time _____

Why am I eating this snack?

_____

Time _____

Why am I eating this snack?

_____

Water 🌢 8oz ◯ ◯ ◯ ◯ ◯ ◯ ◯

Beverages

_____

_____

Cravings / Responses

_____

_____

Activity / Exercise

_____

_____

How to make tomorrow better

_____

_____

_____

_____

I am so proud of myself today because I...

_____

_____

_____

_____

Date	Day of Week	Weight

Breakfast

Time _____   Rate your Hunger 1-10 _____

_____

_____

Lunch

Time _____   Rate your Hunger 1-10 _____

_____

_____

Dinner

Time _____   Rate your Hunger 1-10 _____

_____

_____

Snacks

Time _____

Why am I eating this snack?

_____

Time _____

Why am I eating this snack?

_____

Water ⬤ 8oz   ◯ ◯ ◯ ◯ ◯ ◯ ◯ ◯

Beverages

_____

_____

Cravings / Responses

_____

_____

Activity / Exercise

_____

_____

How to make tomorrow better

_____

_____

_____

_____

I am so proud of myself today because I...

_____

_____

_____

_____

Date	Day of Week	Weight

Breakfast

Time _____   Rate your Hunger 1-10 _____

_____

_____

Lunch

Time _____   Rate your Hunger 1-10 _____

_____

_____

Dinner

Time _____   Rate your Hunger 1-10 _____

_____

_____

Snacks

Time _____

Why am I eating this snack?

_____

Time _____

Why am I eating this snack?

_____

Water ⬦ 8oz ◯ ◯ ◯ ◯ ◯ ◯ ◯

Beverages

_____

_____

Cravings / Responses

_____

_____

Activity / Exercise

_____

_____

How to make tomorrow better

_____

_____

_____

_____

I am so proud of myself today because I...

_____

_____

_____

_____

Date	Day of Week	Weight

Breakfast

Time _____   Rate your Hunger 1-10 _____

_____

_____

Lunch

Time _____   Rate your Hunger 1-10 _____

_____

_____

Dinner

Time _____   Rate your Hunger 1-10 _____

_____

_____

Snacks

Time _____

Why am I eating this snack?

_____

Time _____

Why am I eating this snack?

_____

Water 🜄 8oz ◯ ◯ ◯ ◯ ◯ ◯ ◯

Beverages

_____

_____

Cravings / Responses

_____

_____

Activity / Exercise

_____

_____

How to make tomorrow better

_____

_____

_____

_____

I am so proud of myself today because I...

_____

_____

_____

_____

Date	Day of Week	Weight

Breakfast

Time _____   Rate your Hunger 1-10 _____

_____

_____

Lunch

Time _____   Rate your Hunger 1-10 _____

_____

_____

Dinner

Time _____   Rate your Hunger 1-10 _____

_____

_____

Snacks

Time _____

Why am I eating this snack?

_____

Time _____

Why am I eating this snack?

_____

Water ⬭ 8oz ◯ ◯ ◯ ◯ ◯ ◯ ◯

Beverages

_____

_____

Cravings / Responses

_____

_____

Activity / Exercise

_____

_____

How to make tomorrow better

_____

_____

_____

_____

I am so proud of myself today because I...

_____

_____

_____

_____

Date _____ Day of Week _____ Weight _____

Breakfast

Time _____   Rate your Hunger 1-10 _____

_____

_____

Lunch

Time _____   Rate your Hunger 1-10 _____

_____

_____

Dinner

Time _____   Rate your Hunger 1-10 _____

_____

_____

Snacks

Time _____

Why am I eating this snack?

_____

Time _____

Why am I eating this snack?

_____

Water 🌢 8oz ◯ ◯ ◯ ◯ ◯ ◯ ◯

Beverages

_____

_____

Cravings / Responses

_____

_____

Activity / Exercise

_____

_____

How to make tomorrow better

_____

_____

_____

_____

I am so proud of myself today because I...

_____

_____

_____

_____

Date _____ Day of Week _____ Weight _____

Breakfast

Time _____   Rate your Hunger 1-10 _____

_____

_____

Lunch

Time _____   Rate your Hunger 1-10 _____

_____

_____

Dinner

Time _____   Rate your Hunger 1-10 _____

_____

_____

Snacks

Time _____

Why am I eating this snack?

_____

Time _____

Why am I eating this snack?

_____

Water ⬡ 8oz ◯ ◯ ◯ ◯ ◯ ◯ ◯

Beverages

_____

_____

Cravings / Responses

_____

_____

Activity / Exercise

_____

_____

How to make tomorrow better

_____

_____

_____

_____

I am so proud of myself today because I...

_____

_____

_____

_____

Weekly Progress Tracker

Date

	Measurement	Loss / Gain
Weight		
Left Arm		
Right Arm		
Chest		
Waist		
Hips		
Left Thigh		
Right Thigh		

Weekly Goals

What was my biggest accomplishment for the week?

_____

_____

What new healthy eating choices did I make this week?

_____

_____

What new healthy lifestyle choices did I make this week?

_____

_____

On a scale of 1 - 10 how do I feel about my health and happiness this week? Why do I feel that way?

_____

_____

_____

Rewards for pounds lost

_____

Reasons why being healthy and losing weight matters to me

_____

_____

Date	Day of Week	Weight
⬭	⬭	⬭

Breakfast

Time _____   Rate your Hunger 1-10 _____

_____

_____

Lunch

Time _____   Rate your Hunger 1-10 _____

_____

_____

Dinner

Time _____   Rate your Hunger 1-10 _____

_____

_____

Snacks

Time _____

Why am I eating this snack?

_____

Time _____

Why am I eating this snack?

_____

Water ⬦ 8oz ◯ ◯ ◯ ◯ ◯ ◯ ◯

Beverages

_____

_____

Cravings / Responses

_____

_____

Activity / Exercise

_____

_____

How to make tomorrow better

_____

_____

_____

_____

I am so proud of myself today because I...

_____

_____

_____

_____

Date	Day of Week	Weight

Breakfast

Time _____   Rate your Hunger 1-10 _____

_____

_____

Lunch

Time _____   Rate your Hunger 1-10 _____

_____

_____

Dinner

Time _____   Rate your Hunger 1-10 _____

_____

_____

Snacks

Time _____

Why am I eating this snack?

_____

Time _____

Why am I eating this snack?

_____

Water 🌢 8oz ○ ○ ○ ○ ○ ○ ○ ○

Beverages

_____

_____

Cravings / Responses

_____

_____

Activity / Exercise

_____

_____

How to make tomorrow better

_____

_____

_____

_____

I am so proud of myself today because I...

_____

_____

_____

_____

Date	Day of Week	Weight

Breakfast

Time _____   Rate your Hunger 1-10 _____

_____

_____

Lunch

Time _____   Rate your Hunger 1-10 _____

_____

_____

Dinner

Time _____   Rate your Hunger 1-10 _____

_____

_____

Snacks

Time _____

Why am I eating this snack?

_____

Time _____

Why am I eating this snack?

_____

Water ⬭ 8oz ◯ ◯ ◯ ◯ ◯ ◯ ◯ ◯

Beverages

_____

_____

Cravings / Responses

_____

_____

Activity / Exercise

_____

_____

How to make tomorrow better

_____

_____

_____

_____

I am so proud of myself today because I...

_____

_____

_____

_____

Date _____   Day of Week _____   Weight _____

Breakfast

Time _____   Rate your Hunger 1-10 _____

_____

_____

Lunch

Time _____   Rate your Hunger 1-10 _____

_____

_____

Dinner

Time _____   Rate your Hunger 1-10 _____

_____

_____

Snacks

Time _____

Why am I eating this snack?

_____

Time _____

Why am I eating this snack?

_____

Water ○ 8oz ◯ ◯ ◯ ◯ ◯ ◯ ◯

Beverages

_____

_____

Cravings / Responses

_____

_____

Activity / Exercise

_____

_____

How to make tomorrow better

_____

_____

_____

_____

I am so proud of myself today because I...

_____

_____

_____

_____

Date	Day of Week	Weight

Breakfast

Time _____   Rate your Hunger 1-10 _____

_____

_____

Lunch

Time _____   Rate your Hunger 1-10 _____

_____

_____

Dinner

Time _____   Rate your Hunger 1-10 _____

_____

_____

Snacks

Time _____

Why am I eating this snack?

_____

Time _____

Why am I eating this snack?

_____

Water ⬤ 8oz ◯ ◯ ◯ ◯ ◯ ◯ ◯

Beverages

_____

_____

Cravings / Responses

_____

_____

Activity / Exercise

_____

_____

How to make tomorrow better

_____

_____

_____

_____

I am so proud of myself today because I...

_____

_____

_____

_____

Date	Day of Week	Weight

Breakfast

Time _____   Rate your Hunger 1-10 _____

_____

_____

Lunch

Time _____   Rate your Hunger 1-10 _____

_____

_____

Dinner

Time _____   Rate your Hunger 1-10 _____

_____

_____

Snacks

Time _____

Why am I eating this snack?

_____

Time _____

Why am I eating this snack?

_____

Water ⬤ 8oz ◯ ◯ ◯ ◯ ◯ ◯ ◯

Beverages

_____

_____

Cravings / Responses

_____

_____

Activity / Exercise

_____

_____

How to make tomorrow better

_____

_____

_____

_____

I am so proud of myself today because I...

_____

_____

_____

_____

Date	Day of Week	Weight

Breakfast

Time _____   Rate your Hunger 1-10 _____

_____

_____

Lunch

Time _____   Rate your Hunger 1-10 _____

_____

_____

Dinner

Time _____   Rate your Hunger 1-10 _____

_____

_____

Snacks

Time _____

Why am I eating this snack?

_____

Time _____

Why am I eating this snack?

_____

Water ◌ 8oz ◯ ◯ ◯ ◯ ◯ ◯ ◯

Beverages

_____

_____

Cravings / Responses

_____

_____

Activity / Exercise

_____

_____

How to make tomorrow better

_____

_____

_____

_____

I am so proud of myself today because I...

_____

_____

_____

_____

Weekly Progress Tracker

Date [   ]

	Measurement	Loss / Gain
Weight		
Left Arm		
Right Arm		
Chest		
Waist		
Hips		
Left Thigh		
Right Thigh		

Weekly Goals

What was my biggest accomplishment for the week?

_____

_____

What new healthy eating choices did I make this week?

_____

_____

What new healthy lifestyle choices did I make this week?

_____

_____

On a scale of 1 - 10 how do I feel about my health and happiness this week? Why do I feel that way?

_____

_____

_____

Rewards for pounds lost

_____

Reasons why being healthy and losing weight matters to me

_____

_____

Date	Day of Week	Weight

Breakfast

Time _____   Rate your Hunger 1-10 _____

_____

_____

Lunch

Time _____   Rate your Hunger 1-10 _____

_____

_____

Dinner

Time _____   Rate your Hunger 1-10 _____

_____

_____

Snacks

Time _____

Why am I eating this snack?

_____

Time _____

Why am I eating this snack?

_____

Water ◌ 8oz ◯ ◯ ◯ ◯ ◯ ◯ ◯

Beverages

_____

_____

Cravings / Responses

_____

_____

Activity / Exercise

_____

_____

How to make tomorrow better

_____

_____

_____

_____

I am so proud of myself today because I...

_____

_____

_____

_____

Date	Day of Week	Weight

Breakfast

Time _____   Rate your Hunger 1-10 _____

_____

_____

Lunch

Time _____   Rate your Hunger 1-10 _____

_____

_____

Dinner

Time _____   Rate your Hunger 1-10 _____

_____

_____

Snacks

Time _____

Why am I eating this snack?

_____

Time _____

Why am I eating this snack?

_____

Water ○ 8oz ○ ○ ○ ○ ○ ○ ○ ○

Beverages

_____

_____

Cravings / Responses

_____

_____

Activity / Exercise

_____

_____

How to make tomorrow better

_____

_____

_____

_____

I am so proud of myself today because I...

_____

_____

_____

_____

Date	Day of Week	Weight

Breakfast

Time _____   Rate your Hunger 1-10 _____

_____

_____

Lunch

Time _____   Rate your Hunger 1-10 _____

_____

_____

Dinner

Time _____   Rate your Hunger 1-10 _____

_____

_____

Snacks

Time _____

Why am I eating this snack?

_____

Time _____

Why am I eating this snack?

_____

Water ⬦ 8oz ◯ ◯ ◯ ◯ ◯ ◯ ◯

Beverages

_____

_____

Cravings / Responses

_____

_____

Activity / Exercise

_____

_____

How to make tomorrow better

_____

_____

_____

_____

I am so proud of myself today because I...

_____

_____

_____

_____

Date	Day of Week	Weight

Breakfast

Time _____   Rate your Hunger 1-10 _____

_____

_____

Lunch

Time _____   Rate your Hunger 1-10 _____

_____

_____

Dinner

Time _____   Rate your Hunger 1-10 _____

_____

_____

Snacks

Time _____

Why am I eating this snack?

_____

Time _____

Why am I eating this snack?

_____

Water ○ 8oz ○ ○ ○ ○ ○ ○ ○ ○

Beverages

_____

_____

Cravings / Responses

_____

_____

Activity / Exercise

_____

_____

How to make tomorrow better

_____

_____

_____

_____

I am so proud of myself today because I...

_____

_____

_____

_____

Date	Day of Week	Weight

Breakfast

Time _____   Rate your Hunger 1-10 _____

_____

_____

Lunch

Time _____   Rate your Hunger 1-10 _____

_____

_____

Dinner

Time _____   Rate your Hunger 1-10 _____

_____

_____

Snacks

Time _____

Why am I eating this snack?

_____

Time _____

Why am I eating this snack?

_____

Water ○ 8oz ○ ○ ○ ○ ○ ○ ○ ○

Beverages

_____

_____

Cravings / Responses

_____

_____

Activity / Exercise

_____

_____

How to make tomorrow better

_____

_____

_____

_____

I am so proud of myself today because I...

_____

_____

_____

_____

Date	Day of Week	Weight

Breakfast

Time _____   Rate your Hunger 1-10 _____

_____

_____

Lunch

Time _____   Rate your Hunger 1-10 _____

_____

_____

Dinner

Time _____   Rate your Hunger 1-10 _____

_____

_____

Snacks

Time _____

Why am I eating this snack?

_____

Time _____

Why am I eating this snack?

_____

Water ⬤ 8oz ◯ ◯ ◯ ◯ ◯ ◯ ◯

Beverages

_____

_____

Cravings / Responses

_____

_____

Activity / Exercise

_____

_____

How to make tomorrow better

_____

_____

_____

_____

I am so proud of myself today because I...

_____

_____

_____

_____

Date _____ Day of Week _____ Weight _____

Breakfast

Time _____   Rate your Hunger 1-10 _____

_____

_____

Lunch

Time _____   Rate your Hunger 1-10 _____

_____

_____

Dinner

Time _____   Rate your Hunger 1-10 _____

_____

_____

Snacks

Time _____

Why am I eating this snack?

_____

Time _____

Why am I eating this snack?

_____

Water ○ 8oz ◯ ◯ ◯ ◯ ◯ ◯ ◯

Beverages

_____

_____

Cravings / Responses

_____

_____

Activity / Exercise

_____

_____

How to make tomorrow better

_____

_____

_____

_____

I am so proud of myself today because I...

_____

_____

_____

_____

Weekly Progress Tracker

Date

	Measurement	Loss / Gain
Weight		
Left Arm		
Right Arm		
Chest		
Waist		
Hips		
Left Thigh		
Right Thigh		

Weekly Goals

What was my biggest accomplishment for the week?

_____

_____

What new healthy eating choices did I make this week?

_____

_____

What new healthy lifestyle choices did I make this week?

_____

_____

On a scale of 1 - 10 how do I feel about my health and happiness this week? Why do I feel that way?

_____

_____

_____

Rewards for pounds lost

_____

Reasons why being healthy and losing weight matters to me

_____

_____

Date	Day of Week	Weight

Breakfast

Time _____   Rate your Hunger 1-10 _____

_____

_____

Lunch

Time _____   Rate your Hunger 1-10 _____

_____

_____

Dinner

Time _____   Rate your Hunger 1-10 _____

_____

_____

Snacks

Time _____

Why am I eating this snack?

_____

Time _____

Why am I eating this snack?

_____

Water ⬡ 8oz ⭕ ⭕ ⭕ ⭕ ⭕ ⭕ ⭕

Beverages

_____

_____

Cravings / Responses

_____

_____

Activity / Exercise

_____

_____

How to make tomorrow better

_____

_____

_____

_____

I am so proud of myself today because I...

_____

_____

_____

_____

Date	Day of Week	Weight

Breakfast

Time _____   Rate your Hunger 1-10 _____

_____

_____

Lunch

Time _____   Rate your Hunger 1-10 _____

_____

_____

Dinner

Time _____   Rate your Hunger 1-10 _____

_____

_____

Snacks

Time _____

Why am I eating this snack?

_____

Time _____

Why am I eating this snack?

_____

Water ⬭ 8oz ◯ ◯ ◯ ◯ ◯ ◯ ◯

Beverages

_____

_____

Cravings / Responses

_____

_____

Activity / Exercise

_____

_____

How to make tomorrow better

_____

_____

_____

_____

I am so proud of myself today because I...

_____

_____

_____

_____

Date	Day of Week	Weight

Breakfast

Time _____   Rate your Hunger 1-10 _____

_____

_____

Lunch

Time _____   Rate your Hunger 1-10 _____

_____

_____

Dinner

Time _____   Rate your Hunger 1-10 _____

_____

_____

Snacks

Time _____

Why am I eating this snack?

_____

Time _____

Why am I eating this snack?

_____

Water ⬦ 8oz ◯ ◯ ◯ ◯ ◯ ◯ ◯ ◯

Beverages

_____

_____

Cravings / Responses

_____

_____

Activity / Exercise

_____

_____

How to make tomorrow better

_____

_____

_____

_____

I am so proud of myself today because I...

_____

_____

_____

_____

Date	Day of Week	Weight

Breakfast

Time _____   Rate your Hunger 1-10 _____

_____

_____

Lunch

Time _____   Rate your Hunger 1-10 _____

_____

_____

Dinner

Time _____   Rate your Hunger 1-10 _____

_____

_____

Snacks

Time _____

Why am I eating this snack?

_____

Time _____

Why am I eating this snack?

_____

Water ⬭ 8oz ○ ○ ○ ○ ○ ○ ○

Beverages

_____

_____

Cravings / Responses

_____

_____

Activity / Exercise

_____

_____

How to make tomorrow better

_____

_____

_____

_____

I am so proud of myself today because I...

_____

_____

_____

_____

Date	Day of Week	Weight

Breakfast

Time _____   Rate your Hunger 1-10 _____

_____

_____

Lunch

Time _____   Rate your Hunger 1-10 _____

_____

_____

Dinner

Time _____   Rate your Hunger 1-10 _____

_____

_____

Snacks

Time _____

Why am I eating this snack?

_____

Time _____

Why am I eating this snack?

_____

Water ◯ 8oz ◯ ◯ ◯ ◯ ◯ ◯ ◯

Beverages

_____

_____

Cravings / Responses

_____

_____

Activity / Exercise

_____

_____

How to make tomorrow better

_____

_____

_____

_____

I am so proud of myself today because I...

_____

_____

_____

_____

Date	Day of Week	Weight

Breakfast

Time _____   Rate your Hunger 1-10 _____

_____

_____

Lunch

Time _____   Rate your Hunger 1-10 _____

_____

_____

Dinner

Time _____   Rate your Hunger 1-10 _____

_____

_____

Snacks

Time _____

Why am I eating this snack?

_____

Time _____

Why am I eating this snack?

_____

Water ◌ 8oz   ◯ ◯ ◯ ◯ ◯ ◯ ◯ ◯

Beverages

_____

_____

Cravings / Responses

_____

_____

Activity / Exercise

_____

_____

How to make tomorrow better

_____

_____

_____

_____

I am so proud of myself today because I...

_____

_____

_____

_____

Date	Day of Week	Weight

Breakfast

Time _____   Rate your Hunger 1-10 _____

_____

_____

Lunch

Time _____   Rate your Hunger 1-10 _____

_____

_____

Dinner

Time _____   Rate your Hunger 1-10 _____

_____

_____

Snacks

Time _____

Why am I eating this snack?

_____

Time _____

Why am I eating this snack?

_____

Water ⬤ 8oz ◯ ◯ ◯ ◯ ◯ ◯ ◯

Beverages

_____

_____

Cravings / Responses

_____

_____

Activity / Exercise

_____

_____

How to make tomorrow better

_____

_____

_____

_____

I am so proud of myself today because I...

_____

_____

_____

_____

Weekly Progress Tracker

Date [   ]

	Measurement	Loss / Gain
Weight		
Left Arm		
Right Arm		
Chest		
Waist		
Hips		
Left Thigh		
Right Thigh		

Weekly Goals

What was my biggest accomplishment for the week?

_____

_____

What new healthy eating choices did I make this week?

_____

_____

What new healthy lifestyle choices did I make this week?

_____

_____

On a scale of 1 - 10 how do I feel about my health and happiness this week? Why do I feel that way?

_____

_____

_____

Rewards for pounds lost

_____

Reasons why being healthy and losing weight matters to me

_____

_____

Date	Day of Week	Weight

Breakfast

Time _____   Rate your Hunger 1-10 _____

_____

_____

Lunch

Time _____   Rate your Hunger 1-10 _____

_____

_____

Dinner

Time _____   Rate your Hunger 1-10 _____

_____

_____

Snacks

Time _____

Why am I eating this snack?

_____

Time _____

Why am I eating this snack?

_____

Water ⬤ 8oz ◯ ◯ ◯ ◯ ◯ ◯ ◯

Beverages

_____

_____

Cravings / Responses

_____

_____

Activity / Exercise

_____

_____

How to make tomorrow better

_____

_____

_____

_____

I am so proud of myself today because I...

_____

_____

_____

_____

Date	Day of Week	Weight

Breakfast

Time _____   Rate your Hunger 1-10 _____

_____

_____

Lunch

Time _____   Rate your Hunger 1-10 _____

_____

_____

Dinner

Time _____   Rate your Hunger 1-10 _____

_____

_____

Snacks

Time _____

Why am I eating this snack?

_____

Time _____

Why am I eating this snack?

_____

Water ◌ 8oz ○ ○ ○ ○ ○ ○ ○

Beverages

_____

_____

Cravings / Responses

_____

_____

Activity / Exercise

_____

_____

How to make tomorrow better

_____

_____

_____

_____

I am so proud of myself today because I...

_____

_____

_____

_____

Date _____

Day of Week _____

Weight _____

Breakfast

Time _____   Rate your Hunger 1-10 _____

_____

_____

Lunch

Time _____   Rate your Hunger 1-10 _____

_____

_____

Dinner

Time _____   Rate your Hunger 1-10 _____

_____

_____

Snacks

Time _____

Why am I eating this snack?

_____

Time _____

Why am I eating this snack?

_____

Water ⬡ 8oz ◯ ◯ ◯ ◯ ◯ ◯ ◯

Beverages

_____

_____

Cravings / Responses

_____

_____

Activity / Exercise

_____

_____

How to make tomorrow better

_____

_____

_____

_____

I am so proud of myself today because I...

_____

_____

_____

_____

Date	Day of Week	Weight

Breakfast

Time _____   Rate your Hunger 1-10 _____

_____

_____

Lunch

Time _____   Rate your Hunger 1-10 _____

_____

_____

Dinner

Time _____   Rate your Hunger 1-10 _____

_____

_____

Snacks

Time _____

Why am I eating this snack?

_____

Time _____

Why am I eating this snack?

_____

Water ◯ 8oz ◯ ◯ ◯ ◯ ◯ ◯ ◯ ◯

Beverages

_____

_____

Cravings / Responses

_____

_____

Activity / Exercise

_____

_____

How to make tomorrow better

_____

_____

_____

_____

I am so proud of myself today because I...

_____

_____

_____

_____

Date | Day of Week | Weight

( ) | ( ) | ( )

Breakfast

Time _____ Rate your Hunger 1-10 _____

_____

_____

Lunch

Time _____ Rate your Hunger 1-10 _____

_____

_____

Dinner

Time _____ Rate your Hunger 1-10 _____

_____

_____

Snacks

Time _____

Why am I eating this snack?

_____

Time _____

Why am I eating this snack?

_____

Water 🌢 8oz ◯ ◯ ◯ ◯ ◯ ◯ ◯ ◯

Beverages

_____

_____

Cravings / Responses

_____

_____

Activity / Exercise

_____

_____

How to make tomorrow better

_____

_____

_____

_____

I am so proud of myself today because I...

_____

_____

_____

_____

Date	Day of Week	Weight

Breakfast

Time _____   Rate your Hunger 1-10 _____

_____

_____

Lunch

Time _____   Rate your Hunger 1-10 _____

_____

_____

Dinner

Time _____   Rate your Hunger 1-10 _____

_____

_____

Snacks

Time _____

Why am I eating this snack?

_____

Time _____

Why am I eating this snack?

_____

Water 🜄 8oz   ○ ○ ○ ○ ○ ○ ○

Beverages

_____

_____

Cravings / Responses

_____

_____

Activity / Exercise

_____

_____

How to make tomorrow better

_____

_____

_____

_____

I am so proud of myself today because I...

_____

_____

_____

_____

Date	Day of Week	Weight

Breakfast

Time _____   Rate your Hunger 1-10 _____

_____

_____

Lunch

Time _____   Rate your Hunger 1-10 _____

_____

_____

Dinner

Time _____   Rate your Hunger 1-10 _____

_____

_____

Snacks

Time _____

Why am I eating this snack?

_____

Time _____

Why am I eating this snack?

_____

Water ⬭ 8oz ◯ ◯ ◯ ◯ ◯ ◯ ◯ ◯

Beverages

_____

_____

Cravings / Responses

_____

_____

Activity / Exercise

_____

_____

How to make tomorrow better

_____

_____

_____

_____

I am so proud of myself today because I...

_____

_____

_____

_____

Weekly Progress Tracker

Date

	Measurement	Loss / Gain
Weight		
Left Arm		
Right Arm		
Chest		
Waist		
Hips		
Left Thigh		
Right Thigh		

Weekly Goals

What was my biggest accomplishment for the week?

_____

_____

What new healthy eating choices did I make this week?

_____

_____

What new healthy lifestyle choices did I make this week?

_____

_____

On a scale of 1 - 10 how do I feel about my health and happiness this week? Why do I feel that way?

_____

_____

_____

Rewards for pounds lost

_____

Reasons why being healthy and losing weight matters to me

_____

_____

Date	Day of Week	Weight

Breakfast

Time _____   Rate your Hunger 1-10 _____

_____

_____

Lunch

Time _____   Rate your Hunger 1-10 _____

_____

_____

Dinner

Time _____   Rate your Hunger 1-10 _____

_____

_____

Snacks

Time _____

Why am I eating this snack?

_____

Time _____

Why am I eating this snack?

_____

Water ⬡ 8oz ◯ ◯ ◯ ◯ ◯ ◯ ◯

Beverages

_____

_____

Cravings / Responses

_____

_____

Activity / Exercise

_____

_____

How to make tomorrow better

_____

_____

_____

_____

I am so proud of myself today because I...

_____

_____

_____

_____

Date	Day of Week	Weight

Breakfast

Time _____   Rate your Hunger 1-10 _____

_____

_____

Lunch

Time _____   Rate your Hunger 1-10 _____

_____

_____

Dinner

Time _____   Rate your Hunger 1-10 _____

_____

_____

Snacks

Time _____

Why am I eating this snack?

_____

Time _____

Why am I eating this snack?

_____

Water ⬦ 8oz ◯ ◯ ◯ ◯ ◯ ◯ ◯ ◯

Beverages

_____

_____

Cravings / Responses

_____

_____

Activity / Exercise

_____

_____

How to make tomorrow better

_____

_____

_____

_____

I am so proud of myself today because I...

_____

_____

_____

_____

Date	Day of Week	Weight

Breakfast

Time _____   Rate your Hunger 1-10 _____

_____

_____

Lunch

Time _____   Rate your Hunger 1-10 _____

_____

_____

Dinner

Time _____   Rate your Hunger 1-10 _____

_____

_____

Snacks

Time _____

Why am I eating this snack?

_____

Time _____

Why am I eating this snack?

_____

Water ⬭ 8oz ◯ ◯ ◯ ◯ ◯ ◯ ◯ ◯

Beverages

_____

_____

Cravings / Responses

_____

_____

Activity / Exercise

_____

_____

How to make tomorrow better

_____

_____

_____

_____

I am so proud of myself today because I...

_____

_____

_____

_____

Date	Day of Week	Weight

Breakfast

Time _____   Rate your Hunger 1-10 _____

_____

_____

Lunch

Time _____   Rate your Hunger 1-10 _____

_____

_____

Dinner

Time _____   Rate your Hunger 1-10 _____

_____

_____

Snacks

Time _____

Why am I eating this snack?

_____

Time _____

Why am I eating this snack?

_____

Water ⬭ 8oz ◯ ◯ ◯ ◯ ◯ ◯ ◯ ◯

Beverages

_____

_____

Cravings / Responses

_____

_____

Activity / Exercise

_____

_____

How to make tomorrow better

_____

_____

_____

_____

I am so proud of myself today because I...

_____

_____

_____

_____

Date

Day of Week

Weight

Breakfast

Time _____

Rate your Hunger 1-10 _____

_____

_____

Lunch

Time _____

Rate your Hunger 1-10 _____

_____

_____

Dinner

Time _____

Rate your Hunger 1-10 _____

_____

_____

Snacks

Time _____

Why am I eating this snack?

_____

Time _____

Why am I eating this snack?

_____

Water ◯ 8oz ◯ ◯ ◯ ◯ ◯ ◯ ◯

Beverages

_____

_____

Cravings / Responses

_____

_____

Activity / Exercise

_____

_____

How to make tomorrow better

_____

_____

_____

_____

I am so proud of myself today because I...

_____

_____

_____

_____

Date	Day of Week	Weight

Breakfast

Time _____   Rate your Hunger 1-10 _____

_____

_____

Lunch

Time _____   Rate your Hunger 1-10 _____

_____

_____

Dinner

Time _____   Rate your Hunger 1-10 _____

_____

_____

Snacks

Time _____

Why am I eating this snack?

_____

Time _____

Why am I eating this snack?

_____

Water ⬦ 8oz   ◯ ◯ ◯ ◯ ◯ ◯ ◯ ◯

Beverages

_____

_____

Cravings / Responses

_____

_____

Activity / Exercise

_____

_____

How to make tomorrow better

_____

_____

_____

_____

I am so proud of myself today because I...

_____

_____

_____

_____

Date	Day of Week	Weight

Breakfast

Time _____   Rate your Hunger 1-10 _____

_____

_____

Lunch

Time _____   Rate your Hunger 1-10 _____

_____

_____

Dinner

Time _____   Rate your Hunger 1-10 _____

_____

_____

Snacks

Time _____

Why am I eating this snack?

_____

Time _____

Why am I eating this snack?

_____

Water ⬡ 8oz ◯ ◯ ◯ ◯ ◯ ◯ ◯

Beverages

_____

_____

Cravings / Responses

_____

_____

Activity / Exercise

_____

_____

How to make tomorrow better

_____

_____

_____

_____

I am so proud of myself today because I...

_____

_____

_____

_____

Weekly Progress Tracker

Date _____

	Measurement	Loss / Gain
Weight		
Left Arm		
Right Arm		
Chest		
Waist		
Hips		
Left Thigh		
Right Thigh		

Weekly Goals

What was my biggest accomplishment for the week?

_____

_____

What new healthy eating choices did I make this week?

_____

_____

What new healthy lifestyle choices did I make this week?

_____

_____

On a scale of 1 - 10 how do I feel about my health and happiness this week? Why do I feel that way?

_____

_____

_____

Rewards for pounds lost

_____

Reasons why being healthy and losing weight matters to me

_____

_____

Date	Day of Week	Weight

Breakfast

Time _____   Rate your Hunger 1-10 _____

_____

_____

Lunch

Time _____   Rate your Hunger 1-10 _____

_____

_____

Dinner

Time _____   Rate your Hunger 1-10 _____

_____

_____

Snacks

Time _____

Why am I eating this snack?

_____

Time _____

Why am I eating this snack?

_____

Water ⬭ 8oz ◯ ◯ ◯ ◯ ◯ ◯ ◯ ◯

Beverages

_____

_____

Cravings / Responses

_____

_____

Activity / Exercise

_____

_____

How to make tomorrow better

_____

_____

_____

_____

I am so proud of myself today because I...

_____

_____

_____

_____

Date	Day of Week	Weight

Breakfast

Time _____   Rate your Hunger 1-10 _____

_____

_____

Lunch

Time _____   Rate your Hunger 1-10 _____

_____

_____

Dinner

Time _____   Rate your Hunger 1-10 _____

_____

_____

Snacks

Time _____

Why am I eating this snack?

_____

Time _____

Why am I eating this snack?

_____

Water ⬦ 8oz   ○ ○ ○ ○ ○ ○ ○ ○

Beverages

_____

_____

Cravings / Responses

_____

_____

Activity / Exercise

_____

_____

How to make tomorrow better

_____

_____

_____

_____

I am so proud of myself today because I...

_____

_____

_____

_____

Date	Day of Week	Weight
( )	( )	( )

Breakfast

Time _____   Rate your Hunger 1-10 _____

_____

_____

Lunch

Time _____   Rate your Hunger 1-10 _____

_____

_____

Dinner

Time _____   Rate your Hunger 1-10 _____

_____

_____

Snacks

Time _____

Why am I eating this snack?

_____

Time _____

Why am I eating this snack?

_____

Water ⬦ 8oz ◯ ◯ ◯ ◯ ◯ ◯ ◯ ◯

Beverages

_____

_____

Cravings / Responses

_____

_____

Activity / Exercise

_____

_____

How to make tomorrow better

_____

_____

_____

_____

I am so proud of myself today because I...

_____

_____

_____

_____

Date   Day of Week   Weight

Breakfast

Time _____   Rate your Hunger 1-10 _____

_____

_____

Lunch

Time _____   Rate your Hunger 1-10 _____

_____

_____

Dinner

Time _____   Rate your Hunger 1-10 _____

_____

_____

Snacks

Time _____

Why am I eating this snack?

_____

Time _____

Why am I eating this snack?

_____

Water ⬭ 8oz ⭕ ⭕ ⭕ ⭕ ⭕ ⭕ ⭕ ⭕

Beverages

_____

_____

Cravings / Responses

_____

_____

Activity / Exercise

_____

_____

How to make tomorrow better

_____

_____

_____

_____

I am so proud of myself today because I...

_____

_____

_____

_____

Date	Day of Week	Weight

Breakfast

Time _____   Rate your Hunger 1-10 _____

_____

_____

Lunch

Time _____   Rate your Hunger 1-10 _____

_____

_____

Dinner

Time _____   Rate your Hunger 1-10 _____

_____

_____

Snacks

Time _____

Why am I eating this snack?

_____

Time _____

Why am I eating this snack?

_____

Water ⬭ 8oz ◯ ◯ ◯ ◯ ◯ ◯ ◯

Beverages

_____

_____

Cravings / Responses

_____

_____

Activity / Exercise

_____

_____

How to make tomorrow better

_____

_____

_____

_____

I am so proud of myself today because I...

_____

_____

_____

_____

Date	Day of Week	Weight

Breakfast

Time _____   Rate your Hunger 1-10 _____

_____

_____

Lunch

Time _____   Rate your Hunger 1-10 _____

_____

_____

Dinner

Time _____   Rate your Hunger 1-10 _____

_____

_____

Snacks

Time _____

Why am I eating this snack?

_____

Time _____

Why am I eating this snack?

_____

Water 🜄 8oz ○ ○ ○ ○ ○ ○ ○ ○

Beverages

_____

_____

Cravings / Responses

_____

_____

Activity / Exercise

_____

_____

How to make tomorrow better

_____

_____

_____

_____

I am so proud of myself today because I...

_____

_____

_____

_____

Date   Day of Week   Weight

Breakfast

Time _____   Rate your Hunger 1-10 _____

_____

_____

Lunch

Time _____   Rate your Hunger 1-10 _____

_____

_____

Dinner

Time _____   Rate your Hunger 1-10 _____

_____

_____

Snacks

Time _____

Why am I eating this snack?

_____

Time _____

Why am I eating this snack?

_____

Water ○ 8oz   ○ ○ ○ ○ ○ ○ ○ ○

Beverages

_____

_____

Cravings / Responses

_____

_____

Activity / Exercise

_____

_____

How to make tomorrow better

_____

_____

_____

_____

I am so proud of myself today because I...

_____

_____

_____

_____

Weekly Progress Tracker

Date [   ]

	Measurement	Loss / Gain
Weight		
Left Arm		
Right Arm		
Chest		
Waist		
Hips		
Left Thigh		
Right Thigh		

Weekly Goals

What was my biggest accomplishment for the week?

_____

_____

What new healthy eating choices did I make this week?

_____

_____

What new healthy lifestyle choices did I make this week?

_____

_____

On a scale of 1 - 10 how do I feel about my health and happiness this week? Why do I feel that way?

_____

_____

_____

Rewards for pounds lost

_____

Reasons why being healthy and losing weight matters to me

_____

_____

Date	Day of Week	Weight
( )	( )	( )

Breakfast

Time _____   Rate your Hunger 1-10 _____

_____

_____

Lunch

Time _____   Rate your Hunger 1-10 _____

_____

_____

Dinner

Time _____   Rate your Hunger 1-10 _____

_____

_____

Snacks

Time _____

Why am I eating this snack?

_____

Time _____

Why am I eating this snack?

_____

Water ⬡ 8oz ◯ ◯ ◯ ◯ ◯ ◯ ◯ ◯

Beverages

_____

_____

Cravings / Responses

_____

_____

Activity / Exercise

_____

_____

How to make tomorrow better

_____

_____

_____

_____

I am so proud of myself today because I...

_____

_____

_____

_____

Date	Day of Week	Weight

Breakfast

Time _____   Rate your Hunger 1-10 _____

_____

_____

Lunch

Time _____   Rate your Hunger 1-10 _____

_____

_____

Dinner

Time _____   Rate your Hunger 1-10 _____

_____

_____

Snacks

Time _____

Why am I eating this snack?

_____

Time _____

Why am I eating this snack?

_____

Water ⬫ 8oz ◯ ◯ ◯ ◯ ◯ ◯ ◯ ◯

Beverages

_____

_____

Cravings / Responses

_____

_____

Activity / Exercise

_____

_____

How to make tomorrow better

_____

_____

_____

_____

I am so proud of myself today because I...

_____

_____

_____

_____

Date	Day of Week	Weight

Breakfast

Time _____   Rate your Hunger 1-10 _____

_____

_____

Lunch

Time _____   Rate your Hunger 1-10 _____

_____

_____

Dinner

Time _____   Rate your Hunger 1-10 _____

_____

_____

Snacks

Time _____

Why am I eating this snack?

_____

Time _____

Why am I eating this snack?

_____

Water ⬭ 8oz ◯ ◯ ◯ ◯ ◯ ◯ ◯ ◯

Beverages

_____

_____

Cravings / Responses

_____

_____

Activity / Exercise

_____

_____

How to make tomorrow better

_____

_____

_____

_____

I am so proud of myself today because I...

_____

_____

_____

_____

Date	Day of Week	Weight

Breakfast

Time _____   Rate your Hunger 1-10 _____

_____

_____

Lunch

Time _____   Rate your Hunger 1-10 _____

_____

_____

Dinner

Time _____   Rate your Hunger 1-10 _____

_____

_____

Snacks

Time _____

Why am I eating this snack?

_____

Time _____

Why am I eating this snack?

_____

Water ○ 8oz ◯ ◯ ◯ ◯ ◯ ◯ ◯

Beverages

_____

_____

Cravings / Responses

_____

_____

Activity / Exercise

_____

_____

How to make tomorrow better

_____

_____

_____

_____

I am so proud of myself today because I...

_____

_____

_____

_____

Date	Day of Week	Weight

Breakfast

Time _____   Rate your Hunger 1-10 _____

_____

_____

Lunch

Time _____   Rate your Hunger 1-10 _____

_____

_____

Dinner

Time _____   Rate your Hunger 1-10 _____

_____

_____

Snacks

Time _____

Why am I eating this snack?

_____

Time _____

Why am I eating this snack?

_____

Water ⬤ 8oz ◯ ◯ ◯ ◯ ◯ ◯ ◯ ◯

Beverages

_____

_____

Cravings / Responses

_____

_____

Activity / Exercise

_____

_____

How to make tomorrow better

_____

_____

_____

_____

I am so proud of myself today because I...

_____

_____

_____

_____

Date	Day of Week	Weight

Breakfast

Time _____   Rate your Hunger 1-10 _____

_____

_____

Lunch

Time _____   Rate your Hunger 1-10 _____

_____

_____

Dinner

Time _____   Rate your Hunger 1-10 _____

_____

_____

Snacks

Time _____

Why am I eating this snack?

_____

Time _____

Why am I eating this snack?

_____

Water ◇ 8oz ○ ○ ○ ○ ○ ○ ○ ○

Beverages

_____

_____

Cravings / Responses

_____

_____

Activity / Exercise

_____

_____

How to make tomorrow better

_____

_____

_____

_____

I am so proud of myself today because I...

_____

_____

_____

_____

Date   Day of Week   Weight

Breakfast

Time _____   Rate your Hunger 1-10 _____

_____

_____

Lunch

Time _____   Rate your Hunger 1-10 _____

_____

_____

Dinner

Time _____   Rate your Hunger 1-10 _____

_____

_____

Snacks

Time _____

Why am I eating this snack?

_____

Time _____

Why am I eating this snack?

_____

Water ◌ 8oz   ◯ ◯ ◯ ◯ ◯ ◯ ◯

Beverages

_____

_____

Cravings / Responses

_____

_____

Activity / Exercise

_____

_____

How to make tomorrow better

_____

_____

_____

_____

I am so proud of myself today because I...

_____

_____

_____

_____

Made in the USA
Coppell, TX
23 September 2020